I0435563

Nature's Fitness24

Progressing in fitness lifestyle

- *Basic nutrition*

- *Weight loss and long term easy maintenance*

- *Strength workout for men*

- *Body sculpture workouts for ladies*

- *Healthier home cooking tips*

Nature'sFITNESS24®

Ever noticed when people fall sick to preventable diseases like diabetes, renal (kidney) or cardiac (heart) they become more committed to nutritional health?

Did you know many of us who are on regular free choice diet do not have to wait for dare situation in order to commit to fitness healthier lifestyle?

Have you fallen for quick fix weight loss programs and cover images that promise results only to end up separating you much further from fitness reality?

Due to industrialization and commercial interests, we can fall into a cycle of commercial products trials, promotions and excessive workout. But the nature in you is much stronger than the world system would like you to believe. It all begins with awareness.

The following is a dynamic awareness coaching that can be adjusted to suite your fitness level. This is a proactive coaching packed with knowledge and skill set that will empower you to make nutrition and workout progress.

The coaching includes basic nutrition, overcoming fitness limitations, weight loss and basic cooking.

Joel Mbaire: CDM, CFPP AND CERTIFIED INSTRUCTOR

Nature'sFITNESS24®

Copyrights by Joel Mbaire

Email: naturesfitness24@gmail.com

Table of contents

Chapter 1

Personal Nutrition

As a Chef I assumed I was healthy by just being part of preparing and tasting gourmet meals during production process. I never scheduled for meals and would eat only when I became very hungry. Depending on the company's business of the month and tourism season; I became fairly skinny in one month and my waist and bottom embarrassingly ballooned the following month.

I later joined healthcare industry in the dietary services. Part of my job involved weight and nutritional care plan for patients. This is where I realized how lifestyle choices can indeed waste life.

I served skinny, overweight, old, rich, poor, believers, educated and all kinds of professionals going through strict food restriction while nursing acute and some permanent health issues resulting from preventable health choices. I also witnessed cases of happy ending with remarkable recovery and discharge.

Over the next years, I dedicated my time to practice and learn more about diet and fitness in my everyday life. I realized that even though I had studied nutrition course in school, my focus was only on passing the exams and to serve others in my career path without living it. I was surprised at how little I personally applied what I had learnt.

During this journey, I listened to people who wanted to lose weight and some who had done it before but gained it back.

Like in my case, a common problem was not lack of but the application of the knowledge into their everyday life. This further exposed them into trying different weight loss programs that were hard to maintain on a long term basis despite the initial success.

I was happy to go through the basic nutrition topic one more time but this time for me. Once personalized, I use diet as a tool with ease to lose weight, add weight or support any fitness program that I want to implement; from running marathons to intermediate strength building with success. Today I encourage you to personalize the topics outlined in this book.

Nutrition For weight loss and fitness

Nutrition: Nutrition is a process by which we consume food and drink .The process include how food and drinks are broken down and used inside our body to sustain life.

Meal: Meal describes general times when nutrients are consumed. The common meals times are breakfast, lunch, dinner and snack times.

Diet: Diet is a meal that has a goal .According to USDA dietary guideline, a healthful diet is food and drink that helps to achieve and maintain a healthy weight, reduce risk of diseases and promote overall health.

Special diet: Special diet is food and drinks that have been altered by increasing or reducing on some nutrients in order to meet certain goals. Examples of special diets are weight loss diet, children diet, senior adult diet and weight lifting diet.

Restricted diet: Restricted diet is food and drinks that are served according to doctors or clinical health workers directions. Examples of medical restricted diets are diabetic, renal (kidney), cardiac (heart) and therapeutic diets.

This coaching will focus on weight loss diet and some fitness diets.

Essential nutrients

Depending on what you believe, you may have heard that in the beginning, human being was given dominion over the earth (dry land, water, airspace, and all living things except over other human).To sustain his life, he only gets his food from six essential nutrients.

The Six Essential Nutrients are:

1) **Carbohydrates**
2) **Protein**
3) **Fat**
4) **Vitamins**
5) **Minerals**
6) **Water**

Authority and freedom comes with guidelines, commandments or laws. *There are six guidelines that go alongside each of the six essential nutrients.*

The six Nutritional Guidelines Recommends that we:

- Regularly eat more plants (vegetables and fruits)

- Regularly eat Lean protein (meat, daily, eggs, and legumes)

- Control good carbohydrate serving portions and limit or omit sugar added food

- Control on good oil from plants and limit on solid bad fat (from animals and industrial processed fat)

- Limit on sodium added processed food

- Include sufficient water during meals; snack times, before and after work out.

The above Nutritional Guidelines can also be described using a chart known as food pyramid.

Let us briefly learn how each guideline features in weight loss and fitness goals.

Essential Nutrient: Vitamin

Guideline: Regularly eat more plants (vegetables, and fruit)

Introduction

Green, leafy parts of plants are rich in vitamins. We need Vitamins even though they do not provide energy directly. Our bodies need Vitamins to process energy and optimize metabolism (body functions).

Vitamins are organic (part of living things). Therefore, they can break down (spoil or decay) and lose vitamins. They can also break down through overcooking or prolonged open storage.

To slow down this natural decay and loss of health giving vitamins, fresh vegetables, whole fruits and cut fruits should be stored in the refrigerator or eaten promptly. For the same purpose, vegetables need to be cooked lightly or eaten raw.

Vitamin in fitness programs

Raw vegetables: When eating raw vegetables, choose simple mixed salads that do not require much preparation.

Cooked vegetables: Avoid overcooking vegetables.

> *For weight loss,_vegetables are the primary source of vitamins and fiber; eat vegetables regularly and_increase the serving portion during meals.*

Fruits: Choose a variety of fresh fruits with green and bright colors. Think of rainbow. Eat single fruit, fruit salad, fruit juice and smoothies. Fruits are rich with good carbohydrates, fiber and vitamins.

> *For weight loss,* ***fruits are not the primary source of vitamins,*** *eat fruits regularly but* ***reduce*** *the serving portion.*

Fruit Smoothies and larger portion of fruit salad can be enjoyed occasionally to boost vitamins and energy when recovering from days of high volume exercises or as a healthy treat .The best time to enjoy this treat is during breakfast and lunchtime when soon this ready energy can be put to work.

Unless we are interested in learning the fascinating work of vitamins; or unless we are addressing a particular health issue, it is not a requirement for a fitness participant to know what each particular vitamin does in the body. The important part is to follow the general guideline.

Essential Nutrient: Protein

Guideline: Regularly eat Lean protein (meat, daily, egg, and legume)

Introduction

Protein provides the building materials for growth, repair and maintenance. Protein also contains unavoidable energy. Protein generates 4 calories per gram (same as carbohydrates).

- Some rich Sources of protein are **meats**: chicken, beef, goat, lamb, pork and fish.

- Other rich sources are **non meat**: eggs, milk, yogurt, and legume (bean family)

Protein in fitness programs

Choose lean meat or trim off the excess fat .The National Academy of Sciences (NAS) recommends 56 grams of protein for an adult male per day and 46 grams for a woman; High volume and full time athlete need 50% or more protein per day

The following are common protein measurements (average). Whole egg contain 6g of protein, white egg 3.4g, cup of milk 8g, 4oz (half a cup) chicken breast 29g, medium chicken drumstick 13g, small (beef, pork and goat) weighing 3 oz or 85 grams contain about 20g to 25 g and tilapia 3 oz provides 23g. I cup cooked green gram (ndengu) 14g and cooked beans 15g.It is important to know that other food though not rich in protein also contributes some protein.

Note: The goal of weight loss is to lose fat while maintaining and improving healthy muscles and body repair.

> *For weight loss program you do not cut your lean protein serving. You need it for repair and maintenance.*

Essential Nutrient: Fat

Guideline: Control on clean oil from plants and Limit on bad Solid fat (from animals and industrial processed food)

Introduction

Fat plays a vital role in the body including insulation and energy production when we run out of available energy .Fat also helps the body to absorb some vitamins and more. We can group fat into good and bad fat.

Good oil

This is good and clean oil from plants and fish (Unsaturated fat). Examples of clean oils are olive oil, corn oil, soy bean oil, sun flower, fish oil and avocado oil. Whole grain and nuts like maize, brown rice peanut and cashew has clean oil.

> *For weight loss and other fitness programs whole grains like brown rice, Maize, roast peanuts, cashews, avocados, cooking vegetable oil, salad dressing are some of the primary sources of **the little amount** of good oil needed in meals.*

Bad Fat and oil

This is (saturated fats) like fatty meats. The fat is mostly found in hamburgers and sausages; lard, ghee and margarine .This type of fat raises bad cholesterol levels.

This group also consists of semi solid oil (Tran's fat oil). Tran's fat are industrial fats like semi solid Shortening and margarine and are also considered bad fat. Deep Fried foods and baked pastries contain Trans-fat.

Both saturated fat and Trans-fat raises bad cholesterol levels.

For weight loss and all other fitness programs, Limiting or omitting both saturated and Trans fat reduces both unnecessary weight gain and cholesterol impurities. (Use small amount to cook if you have no other choice)

Introduction to Cholesterol

Cholesterol is a substance that our body need for special functions. But our Liver makes almost all its own cholesterol as needed. Animals also make their own cholesterol for their own use. Our goal is to get protein and other good nutrients from animals which we don't have. We do not need added cholesterol from animals.

Cholesterol from animal will therefore come as an impurity wrapped up within solid fat. Extra cholesterol is dumped inside the veins and artery walls; and may cause high blood pressure. Our body can eliminate limited bad cholesterol as long as we limit bad oils and continue following the clean oil as per the guideline.

Cholesterol in weight loss and fitness

According to Australian eat for health educator's guidelines, high cholesterol elevates the risks of high blood pressure. High cholesterol added into a weak body elevates those risks to even higher levels.

Exercise strengthens the heart, lungs and promotes healthy weight. Combination of *a healthy diet, exercise and healthy weight* enables the body to attain the overall vitality, physical wellness and reduces some health risks.

Essential Nutrient: Carbohydrates

Guideline: Control on good carbohydrates food portion and Limit or omit empty carbohydrate food

Introduction

Carbohydrate is a broad name for sugar. After Carbohydrate is digested, our hungry body absorbs carbohydrates in the form of Glucose. *Carbohydrate is the primary source of energy (calories).* We can group carbohydrates into 3 groups.

Carbohydrate Group A

This is good carbohydrates and includes complex sugars from whole grains like whole maize, sorghum, millet, brown rice and whole wheat products like brown bread. Tubers and roots like potatoes, arrow roots and fruits belong to this group. Foods in this group are rich in carbohydrates and fiber. This type of carbohydrate contains **energy that is released gradually** and delays hunger. *For weight loss choose some of the whole foods regularly but reduce the portion size.*

Carbohydrate Group B

This is good carbohydrates; it includes white starch like ugali, white chapatti, white bread, white spaghetti and white rice. Carbohydrate in this group has less or no fiber. This type of carbohydrates contains **energy that is released much faster** and causes hunger. *For weight loss reduce the serving portion when eating from this group and increase the serving portion of vegetables like spinach.* Choose from this group however when in need of immediate energy like when fueling an hour or two before running, fueling days before a long run (carb loading) ,and during heavy physical work .

Carbohydrate Group C

This group of carbohydrate consists of pure sugars or concentrates loaded in sweetened juices, sodas, cakes, donuts, coated pastries, and ice cream. For this group fiber is missing.

Other carbohydrates in this group are processed foods like popcorn and bagged chips. Tran's fat and extra sodium are also added into the product. Products in this group are more likely to be eaten alone and not within a meal which promotes cravings and weight gain. For this reason food in group C are referred to as empty calories or junk food.

Carbohydrates in group C contain excessive **energy that is released immediately and hunger felt sooner.** *This group of carbohydrates contributes to weight gain and promotes teeth decay. For weight loss and overall health, limit or omit food in group C.*

*Note: Carbohydrate is the primary source of your energy (calories). But, for weight loss, your body fat provides an additional source of energy for doing cardio exercise and work resulting into weight loss. Regularly eat carbohydrates from group **A and B** but reduce on the serving portion in meals. For weight loss and overall health, limit or omit food in group C.*

Fiber

Fiber comes from all parts of plants: tubers, roots, stem, leaves, flowers and seeds. *Legumes* are seeds like beans and are rich in protein. *Grains* are also seeds from the grass family e.g. Wheat, corn, rice, sorghum and millet and are rich in carbohydrates.

Fiber or roughage is a carbohydrate that has no energy value because our body cannot be able to digest it. But fiber has its place in weight loss and fitness.

The Intestine walls movement (peristaltic wave motion) works smoothly when full than when half empty. Fiber provides this filling or bulk in the intestine without giving us unneeded calories. Lack of fiber can cause constipation which is basically stalled movement.

Fiber also make us feel satisfied and reduces hunger and the urge to eat more calories which make fiber one of the best tool for weight loss and fitness management.

When eating carbohydrates from group B ,increase serving portion of fiber rich vegetables like, spinach, sukumawiki (kale), cabbage, string beans, green pepper (Pilipili hoho),celery ,cauliflower, lettuce, tomatoes, carrots and cucumbers when cooking or when eating raw salad. These items can supplement the fiber which is lacking in group B.

Some combination from group A carbohydrates like mixed beans and maize (githeri), beans and potatoes, Brown rice and beans, brown chapatti or brown breads with spinach or other green vegetables are sometimes regarded as super food and are complete meals. Sweet potatoes and arrow roots are good for breakfast and snacks.

Essential Nutrient: Minerals

Guideline: Limit on sodium added processed food

Minerals are non-decaying inorganic elements (not part of living things) .They are found in the soil and water .They can withstand hot cooking. Plant's roots absorb minerals from soil for their use. We absorb minerals into our body from food and drinks.

For weight loss and fitness programs Sodium Chloride (salt) is one of major factor.

Daily recommended salt- taken *within food* per Salt nutritional sticker is about 1 table spoon per day. *The salt we use while cooking is within safe levels* .Hidden salt in processed foods and soft drinks is what we need to check because they can easily add up past allowed daily limits.

Sodium and blood pressure
Sodium is essential for body fluid balance and for blood pressure and functioning of the nerve system (electrolytes). *Kidney regulates sodium.*

According to US centers for Disease Control and prevention, too much sodium causes fluid retention within the bloodstream *(increases blood volume)* and the risk of high blood pressure- *which can hurt arteries and organs.*

Low sodium happens when the body loses fluids through dehydration (severe vomiting, diarrhea, or heavy sweating). Low sodium increases the risk of low blood pressure (low volume). For dehydration through sweating we shall see ahead how to replenish electrolytes after heavy sweating.

Essential Nutrient: Water

Guideline: Include water during meals, snack time, before and after work out.

- Water is essential and forms the basis of life. All the other 5 nutrients depend on water to carry out their functions. We shall include water throughout the training, as part of meals, snacks and during workouts.

Chapter 2

Weight loss and fitness limitations

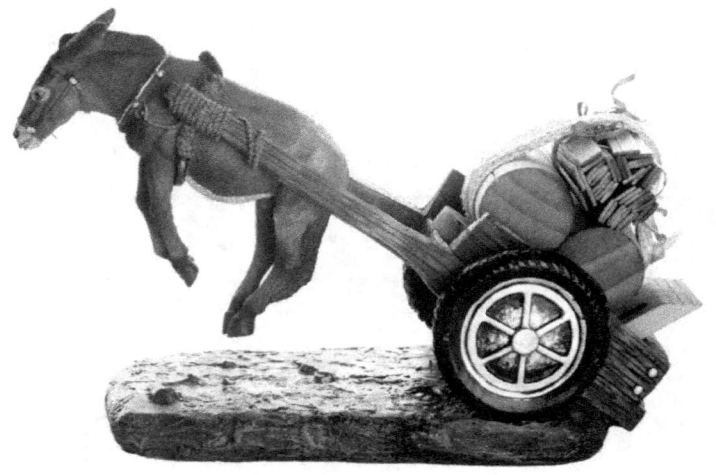

Fitness Limitation: Alcohol

Alcohol is not one of the six essential nutrients; so it's not part of the food supply chain. It introduces energy into the body beyond the recommended food guidelines. Alcohol is processed (metabolized) in the liver. Alcohol is empty calories since it does not contribute other life essential nutrients.

Alcohol also impact nutrition system by temporarily hijacking the liver and mind, which are important nutrition decision-making centers.

Fitness action plan
If your goal is to have fun, include alcohol and maintain healthier body, eat a healthy meal before taking alcohol. The meal should include reduced carbohydrates, lean meat and vegetables. Water is important at any time to avoid dehydration. You should plan to observe the legal limits in order to protect yourself from injury that can further hinder your fitness goals. Consistent full workout is ideal for reversing weight gained.

If your goal is to quit alcohol, self examine the, root cause, advantages and setbacks associated with alcohol. You become what you eat, what you drink and what you do .Alcohol is not food. Alcohol is made from the by-products of decay process of what used to be food.

In her song message *Gia na hinya* (be strong), Julia Lucy warns us not to be like a bull which follows a butcher not knowing it is on the way to get slaughtered. A cruel master, excessive alcohol can kill and we should limit or quit.

Fitness Limitation: Smoking *(cigarette & bhang)*

The Heart needs oxygen rich blood in order to meet increased demands from muscles during exercise and during heavy physical work. Smoking interferes with lungs capability and therefore decreases blood oxygenation. Lack of enough oxygenated blood to sustain heart threshold (maximum heart rate or power), reduces physical endurance in sports and extended heavy duties.

Fitness action plan

If the choice is to quit, like alcohol, the commitment starts from reviewing the root causes, advantages and setback of alcohol and smoking abuse.

Low level of happiness is mostly the root cause of abuse and addiction .Alcohol and smoking tends to temporally fill this gap and helps to lubricate friendship and emotions. Personal influences such as family, relationships, places, idleness, budget and lack of consistent law enforcements facilitates both access and frequency. Is there an alternative?

The hall of fame messenger, Julia Lucy concludes her deliverance song by teaching that unlike the bull; nature has set forth an endless love and happiness covenant; *that if a person runs away or changes ways before they arrive at the destination, that person shall be saved from the blood spill and his/her life purpose will be fulfilled.*

Fitness Limitation: Hunger and over eating

Hunger: Hunger triggers from low blood sugar levels through the stomach and brain mechanism. When the body needs energy, it first reaches for blood sugars and not body fat. If there is no blood sugar, the body initiates hunger pain to tell us it is time to eat healthy food. Eating more calories than we expend will cause weight gain.

Craving: Craving is mind hunger and urge for fast food, sugary food, salty snacks and sugary drinks. It happens when we respond to hunger by eating the wrong food; and therefore not satisfying hunger

Addiction: This is when the body becomes dependant to certain food, drink, substance or certain behavior. Addiction causes you, (soul and mind) to lose control of the body. This causes *excessive* eating, abuse of food and drink; and causes weight gain and other risks.

Starvation: Starvation is part of defense system. It happens when we skip meals. This causes body systems to belief we have a problem getting food and the body naturally starts to rely on body fat for energy.

Hunger and excessive eating action plan

- To avoid starvation, plan your meals in such a way that you do not get too hungry which might cause binge (over) eating.

- Religious fasting is a form of starvation and it's acceptable. The primary goal of spiritual fasting is for you (soul and mind) to train and remind your body that you are in charge and it has to obey your guidelines and believes.

- Fasting and partial fasting can also be utilized for few days occasionally as a process of breaking addictions and habits.

- Partial fasting can be utilized for few days occasionally for weight loss. I prefer this model and I have this protocol:

Eat two meals e.g. breakfast made up of 1 whole egg and 2 or 3 egg whites scrambled with available vegetables), 1 or 2 slices of bread and milk tea, do water all day and eat vegetable or salad and available protein item. - 5 days in a month. Please note that using starvation as a primary strategy for weight loss can result to negative outcomes (ensure you go back to normal meals after planned fasting days)

- To delay and manage hunger, increase the serving portion of fiber rich vegetables. To avoid cravings and addiction, limits or avoids empty carbohydrates from group C. Your tongue can be gradually trained (by you) to get satisfied with less salt and less sugar.

- *Coaching Note: This coaching gravitates toward working adults who can afford meals and adult youth. Starvation and hunger due to famine and due to medical conditions is not the basis of this weight loss and fitness* class.

Fitness Limitation: Lack of Dental Care

Human teeth are tools which enable biting, breaking and grinding food. Teeth are natural jewels, which enhances a smile .Teeth also enhances speech. Teeth are cream whitish in color, which can stain from colored drinks, colored vegetables and, smoking. In addition, teeth are accessory organs, which can suffer infection and decay.

Nature fairly provides each adult with 32 teeth but like other organs and healthy body, the privilege to keep teeth is based on stewardship. Nature allows us to keep more or all teeth when we take good care of them.

Early and regular dental care determines how long each tooth last. Teeth problem is a minefield of health challenges seconded by social implications. Challenges ranges from pain, limited food choices, food texture, food temperature, gum infection, bad breath, choke risk, dental cost, weight loss, and speech challenge.

Some bad groups of bacteria called streptococcus mutans (by J Kilian Clarke in 1924); naturally live within cracks, and around teeth. These bacteria feed on left over sugars and produces acid which erodes teeth under the gum and promotes decay. *Dental is part of fitness for a fact that it is part of digestion system.*

Dental care action plan

The goal in fitness lifestyle is to raise an awareness and emphasis on an individual to make dental care a sustained and highly motivated task. Oral hygiene includes brushing and frosting but in good timing.

Avoid sugary items before bed .Brush teeth or floss after eating sugary items. Flush some water after drinking milk, carbonated sugary soda, coffee, fruit juice and wines to help neutralize sugar and prevent teeth stain.

Dental care also includes visiting the dentist regularly. Dentists have special tools and skills to inspect and offer extra care for an individual tooth. In most countries, dental insurance is outside health insurance.

A fitness participant can revisit and know how much their dental plan covers and actually enjoy the benefits or if they can afford, budget to cover services from out of pocket.

Did you know from 1984 each provincial and district hospital has community oral health workers (COHO).This government (MTC) trained professionals are based in these hospitals with a mandate of taking oral health services to the village level. You can inquire more about how to access these government sponsored services.

Fitness Limitation: Poverty

Poverty at individual level

If you have low source of income, you will be forced to buy the cheapest food that supplies the highest calories regardless of its nutritional properties. The choices could be almost all carbohydrates, all vegetables, all alcohol, or all meat. You will indirectly ration your energy for only basic activities. By natural instincts fitness does not fall under very basic needs (Maslow's hierarchy of needs 1943).

If you have higher resource capabilities but you are unwilling to prioritize nutritional health, you are by natures standards living below the poverty line. No food group by itself can promote optimum health; no resource capability without fitness and diet commitment can promote optimum health. In this case, both groups risks suffering weight loss, weight gain, or impairment.

Poverty by national food policy

The economics of national food security is a wide subject but the trickle down effects is similar around the world. Effects of food insecurity include reduced labor production and less tax income. Less tax income results to social and economic events that lead to high cost of living and high cost of food (inflation).

High cost of living can lead to unhealthy diet choices that can affect the nation.

Common government food policies

Government agencies initiates national food systems by setting minimum dietary guidelines, inspections and aggressive enforcement at public institutions like hospitals, colleges, schools, correctional facilities (jail and rehab); food and drink manufacturing companies, farming, Water ,imported food and alcohol.

Non-governmental Organizations (NGOs) facilitate community food programs through volunteer health professionals, nutritionists, sports athletes, churches, and the media. NGOs target low-income families, poor elderly, poor pregnant, poor disabled *and law abiding refugees.*

NGOs' assistance includes food, milk, subsidized meals, and food awareness, diet education, and counseling, sponsored sports and career training.

For most governments, in this part of the world, the above policies are incomplete. But what happens when government policies are well managed? Would it be the responsibility of the government to feed and to maintain our personal health?

Government food policy and individual healthy choices

Even a well-managed government institution can only do so much to enable the unwilling and to the less informed public consumers. If we personally take charge of our health; the Government policies will merge with our own choices. The law of supply and demands shifts from influencing negative health choices to that of empowering healthy choices within the food chain and support systems.

Each good health decision elicit better society and better public policies: less alcohol results to less accidents and less hospital beds; less (no) bhang results to less anger, and less violence ; improved personal fitness results to less diseases, less stress to medical systems and to family members. The list can go on and on.

In summary, to a large extent, preventable lifestyle diseases and mass poverty are created by the incompetent systems and empowered negatively by her citizen's unhealthy personal lifestyles. The opposite is true; empower yourself at individual level by making a habit of healthy choices and the government systems and policies will by large get empowered positively to respond and match our good choices.

Chapter 3

Fitness Goal: Weight loss

Introduction

Calorie: Energy value we get from food and alcohol is called calorie and energy we burn while working or exercising is also called calorie. Weight gain results from storage of calories or energy that we don't use in form of fat.

Healthy weight (Natural weight)

To know your natural weight you just need your height, age and gender and a healthcare professional or some online calculators can help establish your BMI (Body mass index) and your natural weight. Annual doctors screening can also establish your health status. From this information you can decide how much weight you need to gain, lose or maintain.

If your decision is to lose weight *let us see the relationship between blood sugars, fat and weight loss.*

Relationship between <u>Blood Sugar</u>, <u>Burning Calories,</u> <u>Burning Fat,</u> and <u>Weight Loss</u>

Blood sugar levels

Blood Sugar level is the amount of energy (glucose) present in the blood. Pancreas regulates blood sugar level. Blood sugar is high (we feel high or energetic) after meals, after drinking alcohol, or after taking some drugs.

Blood sugar is normally low (we feel weak), in the morning, after a high performance work out or when we are hungry.

Blood sugar is the ready to use fuel. Unused blood sugar is first stored as reserve energy (glycogen) within the liver and muscles. The rest is converted into fat or weight.

Burning Calories, Burning Fat

The first law of energy (the first law of thermodynamics) states that in the universe, energy cannot be created or destroyed. It can only be transformed, stored or used from one form to another.

In the food chain, plants and meat we eat were once living things that had stored energy within their tissues. When we eat food we inherit energy (calories) that plants and animals had stored in form of carbohydrates, protein and fat.

Weight Loss

Working out to burn fat is giving the body enough reason (stimulate body) to use both blood sugar energy (liquid fuel) and the stored fat (stored excess fuel) resulting into weight loss. *Cardio also known as heart zone or aerobic exercise is the primary exercise for weight loss.*

You have to burn 7000 to 8000 calories, in order to lose 1 Kg. But you do not have to burn all 7 thousands calories same day.

You can run or walk for total 4.8 km and lose about 175 calories (person weighing 74-80 kg) .You do not have to run all 4 miles same day.

Do not procrastinate or quit on your weight loss goals. International CEO's leadership trainer, John .C Maxwell says *"the only guarantee for failure is to stop trying"*

Combination of *cardio exercise, reduced calorie diet and an active lifestyle* is the fastest way to lose and maintain a healthy weight.

But in order to achieve measurable progress in cardio and all other fitness programs, I will now introduce you to fitness basics *known as FITTA guidelines.*

Chapter 4

The FITTA Progress guidelines

FIITA exercise guideline is based on principles of stimulus, response to stimulus and adaptation. In order to be effective, your exercise should follow **FITTA;** whether in cardio, strength or body toning.

FITTA guideline: Frequency, Intensity, Time, Type and Adherence.

Frequency: Frequency is the numbers of exercise session within a week; *3 days to 6 days or every other day.*

Intensity: For the body to improve in fitness, it needs to work harder than it does during normal times. Intensity is the workload for the resistance exercise and the rate of heart beat for the cardio-vascular exercise.

Time: Time is the duration for each session; *ideally 15 to 60 minutes* for fitness ,90 minutes for most sports and over 90 minutes for half and full marathon. Time is also duration when your body is given time to rest and recover from one workout to another.

Type: Type means choosing exercise that you enjoy and progresses your goals e.g. Cardio, weight lifting or sport.

Adherence: Adherence is program's self discipline implying that you must stick to workout program in order for your body to gain results and maintain those results. The protocol of *adherence* must be practiced alongside self control by following the *frequency* guideline to avoid overtraining.

Warm ups, stretching, form & safety

Warm up

To avoid injury, start your workouts with warm ups (about 5min for cardio).Warm up should generally favor the task ahead. If you are preparing to run, warm up on activities, which manipulate lower muscles, legs and core muscles.

If you are preparing to lift weight, warm up on activities that prepare the group of muscles you are about to work on. Warm up by lifting very little or no weight and proceed to lift 3 to 4 sets for that muscle group.

Stretching

Stretching improves your joints, tendons, ligaments, releases tight muscles, improves blood flow and increases flexibility (mobility and range of motion at the joints). Stretching can be done anytime but best after workout or between works.

You should stretch your muscle until you feel controlled tension and not pain at the joint .Your stretch should be a continuous slow movement and not abrupt. Hold your stretch- tension for about 30 seconds

Form & safety

Form is the technique of doing an exercise activity. Performing workout on proper form helps you to avoid injuries and to progress. Bad form fails to engage the target muscles and instead put unnecessary pressure on joints and tendons. Even if you have some success and no pain at the beginning, you increase the risk of injury when you progress to more intense weight and body intensity.

Good form ensures that your back always remain upright and not ached; the core (abdomen area) should be engaged by breathing *in when lowering body or weight* and breathing *out when lifting is entering the peak* .Control lift and do not swing the weight or rush when using body weight. Standard time is 1 second going up and 2sec downwards. Reduce the weight or counts if it feels too heavy *(Even if you have lifted same or heavier before)*.

Exercises of weight lifting with equipments, with body weight and stretching are environments of injury. Do not distracted but focus on the task of workout.

DOMS- Delayed Onset Muscle soreness is the pain that is felt in muscles one to two days after a new exercise is introduced or when you increase workload. Injury pain on the other hand is felt immediately it happens or pain that persists after few days, weeks or months.

Good nutrition helps to prevent a cycle of injuries. Micro-injuries are healed in time and progress is made before the next exercise. Sports gear including sports shoes, clothing, and quality equipment offer comfort, reduce injuries, increases results and save time.

When lifting heavy item including everyday items that are not related to fitness, you must use proper form to avoid injury.

Avoid high risk challenges like HIIT and weight lift if *you are a beginner*. Condition your body for non professional competition for better results.

Take basic safety precaution when outside doing cardio. Study your surroundings and avoid hidden places. Consider getting partners if you are running at night *(dusk to dawn)* within college and within what look like safe neighborhoods during the day *(sunrise to sunset)*.

Common fitness programs:

- Cardio Fitness program *(Fitness For the heart zone)*

- **HIIT and Tempo** Cardio fitness program *(fitness for the heart zone)*

- Strength, body building and endurance program *(Man)*

- Flexibility workout , endurance and toning program *(woman)*

Primary Cardio fitness program *(fitness for the heart zone)*

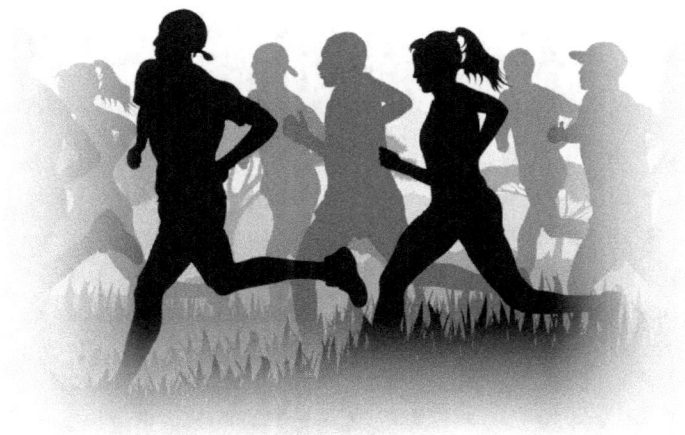

Chapter 5

Cardio Fitness program *(Fitness For the heart zone)*

Introduction

Cardio or aerobic workout is the most complete workout and is the primary exercise for weight loss. Cardio also forms the foundation for all other workout goals including specific sports, weight lifting and muscle toning.

Cardio exercise include, walking, biking, rope jumping, swimming, hiking, Zumba, bollywood, yoga and last but not least circuit training (fast paced repetitive routine).

Energy Fueling

Fueling is eating before an exercise; the food gives your muscles the energy to finish the workout. Fueling does not interfere with the weight loss goal if it's done correctly.

Fueling also protect those who have achieved weight loss goals and are not trying to lose weight.

Energy fueling for moderate cardio below 30 minutes

Energy fueling for weight loss and moderate workout depends on when you ate last and when you intend to eat next. You can decide to eat or not eat if you don't feel hungry.

For moderate cardio, less than 30 minute cardio, you don't have to fuel before exercise and you don't have to replenish fuel after exercise. Your body gets fuel energy from the available blood sugar energy and from the body fat.

Your body therefore can do workout and wait for the next regular meal (of reduced carb and fat) or snack time. The consumption of water before and after a workout is essential.

Energy fueling for cardio 30 to 60 Minutes session

Fueling BEFORE exercise

Eat a carbohydrate snack (banana, an apple, an orange, a piece of bread, fruit juice or a glass of milk) before exercise to meet expected increase in energy demand.

Fueling AFTER a 30 to 60 minutes workout:

For workout recovery we need both carbohydrates snack and protein snack for example, a piece of wheat bread, yoghurt, banana, shake, milk or nuts. We also need to replenish electrolytes after heavy sweating in a hot day (add 1-2 pinch of salt into a glass of water).Replenishing is ideal within an hour after workout.

The consumption of water before and after a workout is essential. *Fuel the same for workout between 60 and 90 minutes but increase the size.*

After your exercise is done you need to go back to your weight loss diet (reduce carb and fat, increase fiber and follow general guidelines discussed earlier) or eat according to your other particular fitness program.

Energy fueling for over 90 minutes (carb loading)

Half marathon is 21 km (13.1 miles) and full marathon is 42 km (26 miles).The primary goal of marathon is not just for weight loss (since weight loss can be achieved and maintained easily at lower level intensity).Non competitive marathon go beyond ordinary goals of fitness and weight loss and challenges your body, your believe and personal limitations.

For those who consider themselves not genetically gifted for running, 21km or 42 km is not easy. Hard work, self discipline and determination can turn a dream which in the beginning appears impossible, to possible .The primary focus for long run is to challenge your personal limitations, other runners are not your competitors; therefore, everyone who starts and finishes is a winner.

We learnt that fasting can be incorporated at the beginning process of breaking addictions and behavior change. Going through pre-marathon training and the actual marathon empowers self confidence to challenge personal limitations.

Train hard few months or weeks before marathon. Progress from running a few miles to running near your goals .Do not just run on flat pathways but include some raised ground and steep levels if possible. .Increase on all your six essential nutrients and get most of your carbohydrates from whole grains. Fuel before practices using pre work out fueling per 60 to 90 minutes.

Few days before actual marathon cut down on exercise and focus on food, stretches and warm ups.

- *One or two days before marathon eat extra carbohydrate meals known as carbohydrate loading or carbo-loading like white pastas, white rice or white bread (white carbohydrates in group A)*

- *Reduce on the serving portion of lean protein, good fat and vegetables.*

- *During the event, an hour or two before running, fuel per 60 minutes pre workout snack and water.*

- *Carry your water and occasionally slow down and take a sip throughout your marathon.*

Extra energy is reserved (loaded) in the body (as glycogen) and will power the completion of a long exercise after blood sugar is depleted. Therefore, energy for long distance is not just from body fat but from loaded carbohydrates and pre workout fueling.

Replenishing AFTER long distance cardio

A prolonged workout lowers blood sugars, electrolytes, water and, 'injures the muscles". Replenishing within an hour after workout should include **electrolytes, carbohydrates, lean protein and water** (a banana plus 1 ½ cup of milk can be good sources).

After marathon, resume your weight loss diet or your particular fitness program and follow FITTA guidelines.

Chapter 6

HIIT (High Intensity Interval Training) **and Tempo Cardio** (fitness for the heart zone)

In regular cardio (with air or aerobic) you run steadily within your heart limits and your level of fitness. If your goal is to cover 2km, you cover this distance with about the same speed. For a beginner, this is hard.

Tempo cardio; alternating between moderate speed, walking and jogging assists you to progress in speed and endurance. In both cases; Tempo and steady cardio, you have enough oxygen to sustain your activity for longer period and to cover your target distance (and you are able to talk).

In HIIT, you push your body to maximum limits and alternate with very moderate intensity to bring back your heart rate to near normal and repeat: *Sprint for 30 seconds and walk or rest for a minute then sprints again and repeat.*

HIIT workout session last less than 20 minutes with the first 5 minutes utilized for warm up. For HIIT your body does not have enough oxygen (anaerobic) to sustain the activity for long (and you can barely talk).

HIIT is the preferred cardio for body builders and experienced athletes. Due to the intensity involved, *HIIT program is not the best exercise for a beginner.*

Chapter 7

Strength, muscles and endurance program (man)

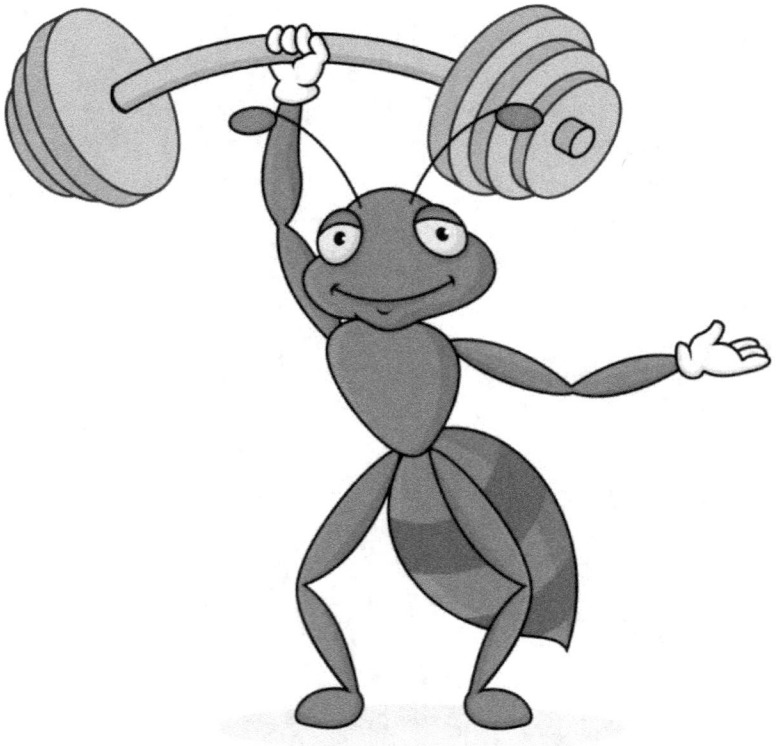

Strength, muscles and endurance program (Man)

Losing weight through cardio is a major goal. After this goal is achieved some people feel it's time to add few muscles to their body structure. Muscles have higher density than fat. Moderate muscles will occupy less space than fat making you appear lean and not thin. They also increase your working strength and you fit well in clothes.

The following topic is about strength workout with a goal of increasing your physical potential of a working man.

Weight lifting goals

If you walk into a gymnasium and start lifting weight up and down; this is known as a rep or repetition. When you stop lifting and rest for a minute or two, you have completed one set of repetition. If you continue lifting and then stop you have completed the second set. The standard number of sets for better result is 3 to 4 sets.

The number of times (reps) you lift in a set will give you different results for that muscle group. If you lift to a count of 6 to 8 reps in a set, you condition your body for strength .If you lift for a count of 10 to 12 reps in a set; you will increase your muscles. If you lift for count of 15 to 20 reps in a set, you will increase muscle endurance (Endurance is the stamina or the ability to keep doing something for a long duration without tiring).

All three choices will give you each of the three benefits to a certain degree; you will just have more of what you work for, according to your genetics and your nutrition.

Your lift will look like this example;

18kg lift 15 rest lift 15 rest; for **endurance.**

18 kg lift 6 rest lift 6 rest; for **strength.**

18kg lift 12 rest lift 12 rest; **for muscles.**

You can mix up between three sets or you can alternate. You can also increase from 3 to 4 sets.

Target 2 to 3 muscle groups in a session *(best results less than 45 min)*.Work each muscle groups once or twice a week

How to determine your beginning strength

Lift weight that is *light enough* not to cause injury but *heavy enough* that it feels difficult to lift more than 6 counts. This is called beginning weight and this is how you determine for each muscle group. When (in a week or two) the weight feels too light it means your body responded well to stimuli and you have made progress.

You can now increase weight (resistance) from one of these three choices. Increase the weight from 18Kg to 20 Kg.; reduce rest time from 1 minute down to 30 seconds or count from 6 to 8. In either case your resistance increment need to be minimal. When you start lifting, you quickly learn how to make your own customized program.

Weight lifting diet

Lifting weight gives your body reasons to grow and you have to provide the building materials. Choose the below meals for weight lifting diet. Fuel with carbohydrate snack like fruit, i.e. banana before workout and replenish with protein for recovery starting within an hour after workout.

- Increase on the serving portion of lean protein in your meals.

- Reduce the serving portion of carbohydrates and Prepare most of your carbohydrates from whole grains and whole grain products (this varies from time to time and depends on your weight goals at the time)

- For protein supplements; use when you cannot access enough protein from food and shouldn't be the primary source of protein.

- Increase on the serving portion of fiber rich vegetables (for vitamins and to manage hunger).

- Increase water intake.

Muscle groups

Your **pushing muscles** are chest, shoulders and triceps (behind upper arm). To progress using your own weight do push- ups *(regular, wide & close)* .To progress using equipments, do dumbbell press and dips.

Your **pulling muscles** are biceps (front upper arms), latissimus dorsi or lats (side-chest under arms) and upper back shoulders. To progress using your own weight, do chin up and pull ups. To progress using equipments do bicep curls for biceps and barbell (or dumbbell) over row.

 Your **core muscles** are Lower back, elector spine, abdomen and legs: To progress using your own weight, do crunches, sit ups, leg raise, running and free squat. To progress using equipments; do barbell squats for lower back, elector spine abdomen and legs.

When lifting, you can reduce on cardio but don't eliminate. You can do cardio twice or three times a week; *just enough to support your primary goals of weight lifting.* You can do HIIT on your weight lifting off day or after your upper body work out days.

Farmers walk is an exercise for the forearm and one of the top exercises in strong man workouts. In this exercise, you carry two heavy items of equal weight, one on each hand. The weight could be a mechanic, construction, farming item or dumbbells.

Move items from point A to B counting for 30 seconds and progress to 60 seconds.

Coaching Note: The strength of a human being remains in the mind and individual talent. The physical work standards coached here is not that of a strong man pulling a bus and uprooting small trees. This is about healthier living, fun and to help us increase on some working physical strength.

Based on those goals we need to be committed but not overly aggressive to a point of using growth hormones *(anabolic steroids)*. If you have other health goals, work with your doctor or a healthcare professional. To begin with, practice form/style for each exercise with little or no weight. *In order to avoid injuries, confirm online how to correctly implement the form and follow FITTA guidelines.*

Chapter 8

Body toning and endurance program (woman)

Body toning or muscle toning is secondary to the primary weight loss goals and endurance cardio. Toning is having low level of fat covering her flexibility lean muscles, her posture and her mobility muscles. You can develop defined body by using your body weight and through stretches.

- For **Core, abdomen and hips do** crunches, sit ups and leg raise .Resistant ball and resistant bands can be incorporated and recommended.
- For Upper **legs *and* elector spine do** body weight lunge and body weight squat. For **side stomach, hips all the way to the ankle do** angled Side Bridge. *Confirm online how to progress on each.*
- Do your toning workout in a slow controlled manner. Take about two seconds on downwards movements and one second on upwards movements. Breathe in when going down and out when going up.
- Stretch different muscles and hold your stretched muscle for 30 sec. Stretch your joints in a controlled manner until you feel slight pinch and not pain.

For each group of toning exercise, choose one or two and do twice a week. Do the exercise for 45 counts in groups of 15 with 2 minutes rest in between. *(Progress slowly. Confirm online how to perform even for those styles which seems obvious).*

An individual's genetic makeup determines which part(s) of the body the extra fat is stored. It could be in the legs, the abdomen, back, shoulders, upper arms, or around the hips.

A weight watcher cannot decide which part of body will lose weight first (unless you go for clinical methods). Just because the desired part of the body appears to have not changed does not mean weight loss or other goals never occurred.

Chapter 9

What is your physical strength level?

Physical work standards

Department of labor; dictionary of social security administration physical exertion requirements classifies physical jobs as **sedentary work, light work, medium work, heavy work and very heavy work.**

Sedentary work: Sedentary work involves occasionally lifting at least 4.5kg. (10 pounds).Most of the job is done while on sitting posture mixed with some walking and some standing .It also involves occasionally moving small weights like pushing a chair, a file and other small tools.

Light work: Light work involves lifting at least 9Kg. (20 pounds) at some points with frequent walking and frequent standing and some sedentary work.

Medium work: Medium work involves lifting at least 22 Kg. (50 pounds) at some points with frequent doing lightweight mixed with some sedentary work

Heavy work: Heavy work involves lifting at least 45Kg. (100 pounds) at some points with frequent doing medium work, mixed with light work and some sedentary.

Very heavy work: Very heavy work involves lifting more than 45 Kg. (100 pounds) at some points with frequent doing heavy work, mixed with medium work, light work and some sedentary work.

Physical work analysis

Due to the use of machines, smart technology and tasks delegation, our physical jobs will continue falling to sedentary and light work.

Some jobs like commercial driving fall under light work for cars and medium work for heavy trucks; but the work is unevenly distributed and the posture is almost fixed. The driver's helper could be doing endurance cardio all day but most of them might not have diet capabilities to support this energy demands *(see poverty at individual level page 30 & fitness limitations)*.

Let's look at another medium work of a nurse. She has to constantly and kindly pick up, pull, push the patients, walk to the patients, walk the patients; and bend to encourage, bend to feed, and tuck the bed and more. Her work is evenly spread and all she needs is good diet and rest time.

In old school farming-whichever one; they used to implement manual work but had access to food in the farm and took breaks under the trees. We cannot turn back the clock; but, we can implement *regular stretch* while working, *regular exercise*, *diet* and *breaks* can fill the balance and help retain that traditional heavy-duty - capabilities of a working man; and mobility and flexibility of an active modern woman.

Unless there is injury, pregnancy, aging, poverty, famine and situation beyond our capabilities, our bodies can remain at their best natural potential. Technology should make us produce more without taking over our natural potential. Per what we have learnt so far you are able regulate food intake and exercise to match different life changing events at work and out of work situations.

Fitness and stress management

Stress is how the mind naturally prepares to respond to daily pressures or illness. Pressures include daily obstacles: workload, work systems, a manager, long working hours, exam, an interview, intense competition or traffic jam.

Life situations could be: financial situation, marriage situation, lack of job, harassment or body weight situation. Stress causes irritability, sleep disturbance and weight gain. Prolonged stress increases production of fat storing hormones (cortisol) which leads to weight gain.

Physical exercise boosts the immune system, increases body performance and improves sleep. According to Mayo clinic, exercise also increases production of body substance *(endorphins)* responsible for raising happiness and lowering stress and pain.

Part 2

Home Cooking Improvement

&

Food protection

Introduction

In part one; we learnt about six life essential nutrients; **carbohydrate, proteins, fats, Vitamins, minerals and water**. We learnt what to eat and what to avoid. We learnt about food portioning and how to utilize diet to support our exercises and work lifestyles.

Food passes through food flow stages: **Farm – Food market – Kitchen - Cooking – Serving Plate**. Nutritional and fitness decisions *practically* happen along this food pathways.

We learnt most foods are organic (part of living thing), and so they can decay (spoil) and lose those life giving nutrients they carry. We don't want to look for life where there is none. *Part two will help us to know how to protect the wholesomeness of the food and to preserve their shelf life.*

Most of us are care providers for children and elderly members in the family. This group requires extra nutritional needs to attend to; the needs are associated with child growth and health maintenance for senior adults.

By a click of a button, we can view or download more than 1000 different ways of cooking any item. Some wise persons once said that many cooks ruin the dish. With many selections, it may be hard to pick what is best for us and flexible enough to cater for fitness and diet needs in the family.

How about if I can coach you on the key elements from what you know; and together we can improve on food flow decision making points and cooking. This coaching is about a few building blocks that can help us to select the best food, how to preserve their shelf life and how to cook for a healthier family.

If you are not directly involved in cooking, this coaching can improve the skills of your house help, your personal chef, or a gift to someone for healthier family.

Chapter 10

Improving on food purchasing skills

In order to comply with nutritional guidelines at each food supply stage (Farm-food market-kitchen-cooking-and plate), remember acronym **ROIS: Reduce** on something **Omit something, improve** on something *(skill or knowledge) and* **Substitute something.**

Menu planning, Purchasing

Have a menu plan for at least 5 days of the week. The 5 days stock does not mean spending much; they may actually be the money saving days.

Buy at least 3 types of meats and one type of bean (lentil, beans or ndengus) Consider buying staple food (rice, flour, dry beans, maize, sugar and potatoes) in bulk. Don't forget to include breakfast and snack options like sweet potatoes arrow roots, breads and healthier cereals.

Reduce or omit

Reduce or omit on the quantity of canned vegetables, canned meat and canned fruits; buy low or no added salt or sugar products. Omit sodas, chips, cookies. Reduce or omit Trans' fat products. Consider more fresh fruits over liquid juice. Compare the price of processed meat and decide if the same price can purchase fresh product. Do processed foods occasionally.

Always go for freshness and brightness on vegetables. Do not buy poor quality vegetables that can go to waste before cooking. Use color to decide freshness and quality. If you have a refrigerator, consider frozen uncooked vegetables;

they are nutritionally as good as fresh. If you don't have a refrigerator, keep perishable food in a cool place.

In the kitchen, cook/use highly perishables like spinach and salads first and plan for less perishables like beans, potatoes, and frozen vegetables toward the end of your week menu. If you find a deal on vegetables like spinach, sukumawiki, and green beans and you want to hold them for more than a week; and you have a freezer; consider blanching them before freezing.

Purchasing International food

You know how to cook most of your staple food or favorite food; you just need to do a few upgrades in order to make them healthier. But once in a while, try some international food and locate their local store. For generations, some countries have guarded their food from cultural erosion.

If you frequently like world celebrated theme foods like Italian, Chinese, French, Indian, Israel, Ethiopian, Morocco and Mexican food, always keep the best of their ingredients or spices they use in almost all their food. It is very hard to buy some of the spices when you need them.

Improving on home kitchen skills

Food Protection

Bacteria are everywhere, from humans (nose, throat, hands, and clothing) and from water and soil. Illness bacterium comes from water and soil and can be passed on to us through food. *Food illness causing bacteria are not many but cannot be seen or smelled. Some other bacteria do not cause illness but they can spoil food.*

Some foods promote bacteria if they have protein, air, water or right environment for growth. All protein rich foods; milk, milk products, poultry, fish, shellfish, soy protein food, cooked beans, soy (tofu), meat, sliced melon, baked potatoes, raw seeds, and raw vegetables can easily support bacterial growth. The following are the three areas we should keep an eye on:

Time: Hold cold food cold. Hold hot food hot. Serve cold food cold, serve hot food hot. Do not keep warm food for more than 6 hours without refrigerating or eating. *(Or keep in a cool place if you don't have a refrigerator).*

Temperature: Avoid undercooked food. Reheat food to a high temperature over 165f (fully hot and not warm). Refrigerate vegetables and fruits after cutting. *(Or keep in a cool place if you don't have a refrigerator).*

Sanitation: wash hands before touching ready to eat food with bare hands. Separate ready to eat food from raw food.

Do not buy dented canned foods. A small dent can let in some air inside the can. This can cause germination of Illness causing bacteria Clostrtridium Botulinum (discovery by Emile Pierre van Ermengem, 1895).

Frozen and refrigerated food

Nutritional value remains intact when fresh or cooked food is frozen. Refrigerated cooked food should be eaten best within 3 days or freeze it. Investing on a freezer is not a waste; money saved from wasted food outweighs the initial expense. In case of power outage, most freezers can hold frozen food for two days without thawing.

Kitchen General Safety

When food reaches boiling point, reduce heat to prevent over boiling. Avoid over filling pots and food containers with food while cooking. Remove pot cover slowly and by lifting sideways to avoid steam scalding hands and face. Use a ladle to pour food to prevent spills and burns.

To avoid burns do not leave cooking ladles hanging on the pot sides or positioned over open flame. Use dry mitts or dry cloth when handling hot utensils; assume pots are hot. Avoid easily shredded, abrasive materials such as steel wool for cleaning utensils. Soak the pots instead and use softer cleaning materials.

Food Wastage

Food spoilage and food waste happens in the food chain during *harvesting, processing, food transportation, in the market stores and consumer's homes.* According to World Food program (WFP) fight for hunger, effects of wasted and spoiled food at consumer level is wasted time to the store, time spent cooking, lost money and loss of life sustaining nutrients.

This training is about health and fitness cooking .The decision and skill set that goes into food preparation; and the self discipline you must have to succeed in fitness lifestyle, are intimately interwoven with that of food waste reduction at individual level and national food policy (see page 31 and 32).

Upgrading diet for children

Children have special needs associated with growing which include developing body mass, strengthening of bones and developing self-independence

Nutrition

Nutritional guidelines for kids are the same as adults. Prepare all six nutrients according to nutritional guidelines .When serving meals and snacks for children;

- *Regularly serve milk or dairy*

- *Serve and encourage them to eat vegetables and fruits.*

- *Serve child appropriate food portion.*

Encourage age appropriate independent tasks (with supervision) to strengthen bones and growth. Include fun in the tasks .Support early child oral care.

Support, encourage kids to be part of the school and community physical activity programs. Diet, exercise and good dental care habits will likely be carried over to adult life.

Upgrading food for senior Adults

Primary aging

Primary aging refers to unavoidable decline in our body system which is influenced by nature. It includes decline in muscle mass, immune system, bone strength, digestion system, endurance and balance. *We are not in charge of primary aging.*

Secondary aging

Secondary aging refers to the current lifestyle and previous unresolved issues added to the primary aging. The factors include nutrition, physical activities, previous accidents, previous work injuries, oral care, smoking habits, alcohol abuse etc.

We are in charge of the secondary factors .We have capabilities to delay or control effects of secondary factors. Aging with complications refers to the effects of secondary aging going out of control.

Nutrition and fitness for secondary aging

The goal is to ensure the body remains in its most natural potential even at the senior age. Due to the weakening bone structure weight increase is to be avoided. Senior Adults diet would look like weight loss diet but with reduced sodium (Salt) thus:

Prepare all six nutrients according to nutritional guidelines .When serving meals and snacks for senior adults;

- *Reduce on carbohydrates serving portion*

- *Serve enough protein*

- *Increase on vegetable serving portion*

- *Reduce salt in food*

Exercise, diet and healthcare professional guidelines at any time in life can *slow the secondary aging progress* and Prolong self-independence. Exercise strengthens lungs; heart functions and muscle strength.

But, as the primary aging advances there is strength and threshold for which the body can endure; appropriate exercises need to be skewed to fit appropriate age group to avoid injuries.

BONUS:

COOKING METHODS

COOKING TIPS

Basic cooking methods

Cooking is divided in to two general methods: **cooking with water or dry cooking.**

Cooking with water

Cooking with water styles are described according to how much water used.

In steaming, very little water is used; heat is reduced to medium after boil and cooking pot covered tight. Steaming is best for vegetables, rice, and fish and as part of recipes. It can be done in oven or on counter stove top.

In pot roast, little water reaching up to ¼ the item is used, heat reduced to medium after boil and cooking pot covered. Rough cut mixed vegetable are added 20 to 30 minutes before meat get ready. Pot roast is best for big joint requiring long slow cooking (2 to 3 hrs) like whole chicken, shoulder or whole leg meat. During serving the meat is sliced, the water has turned in to sauce which is spread over the meat. Skim off floating fat from the sauce using spoon or ladle. Pot roasting can be used in combination of other methods in specific recipes.

In boiling the liquid is bubbling and hot water has fast movement. Vegetables, pasta, grains and legumes are cooked using this method. As general rule items that cook faster like vegetables, pasta, rice and eggs are boiled starting from boiling liquid. Slower cooking items like Potatoes, grains like dry maize, and legumes like dry beans are boiled starting from cold water.

In stewing water is added to just cover the meat and heat is reduced to simmer after it boils; pot covered. You should see few meet pieces not covered with water. Cut mixed vegetables same sizes as meat and add the vegetables 20 to 30 minutes before meat get ready.

In simmering water or stock is brought to boil and then reduced from aggressive boiling to slow moving. Simmering helps your food not break from aggressive boiling and you do not have excessive evaporation.

Dry cooking

In dry cooking the methods are described according to where the dry heat is coming from.

Pan frying: The food item is placed on a hot pan covered with thin oil film. Heat comes from the pan to the item on contact. Items are turned to allow heat contact on both sides. In this method, cuts like steaks and fish fillet cooks within a short time. French speaking, the term *Sautéing* is regarded classy and is preferred when describing pan-frying.

Stir-fry is pan frying meat and then adding vegetables and starch items. In other words protein, vitamin, and carbohydrate sources are all stirred together Chinese style. In this method, a delicious nutrient- packed meal is surprisingly ready within a short time. Stir-fry method is easy and oftentimes a must know in a fitness program.

Broiling is related to grilling. In grilling, heat comes from under, in broiling heat comes from the top and it's usually a selection option on the oven. The item need turning and it's good for fish chicken breast or other non tough meats.

Grilling is using open flame, charcoal grill, gas grill, griddle or other equipment where heat comes from under. Grilling can be done inside but is mostly associated with outside open flame. Barbeque may also refer to grilling or it may refer to the use of barbeque sauce on the meat product.

Roasting is baking where heat come from all sides' .The difference comes from what purpose each term was used. Roasting is baking refereeing to meat and vegetables and grains like roast maize.

Both Roast and grills are highly cherished in Africa. The natural skills, the passion, temporally peace and unity they initiate in a family setting make them also the top choice for greasing friendships, relationship ice breaking, and partly, deal breaking instrument in businesses.

Baking is associated with cakes, pies, pastry and breads. While hot cooking allows for some flexibility when cooking; a more precise measurement is adhered to in bakery due to chemistry involved to raise the dough, baking temperature, emulsifying egg and butter, liquid and sugar factors.

Note: *We learnt in part one that industrial processed food like canned food, sausages, bagged chips, biscuits, pop corns, ice creams etc contain added sodium, saturated fat and Tran's fat and added sugar. Not all industrial food is bad milk flour and yogurt being examples.*

Cooking food has a lot of advantages .Fire; electricity and gas are as a result of human industrial revolution. Therefore keep in mind cooking is food processing and deep frying, cake baking and casserole etc. can be regarded as extensive food processing .Follow the six nutrition guidelines to make food decisions.

COOKING TIPS

Cooking dry Beans

Beans are rich in protein but beans causes stomach upset to most people. Beans contain complex sugar (oligosaccharides) for which our body has no enzymes to digest. This sugar naturally ferments at the lower intestine before removal which causes 'joyful' moments.

Sugar dissolves in water. Our goal is to reduce this sugar to safe levels. By soaking beans in water and letting it sit for 8 to 10 hours or overnight, it allows for most sugars to dissolve .For quick soaking place beans in cold water and heat to boil .Remove from heat and let it sit for 2 hours .Do not reuse the soaking water; rinse the beans and use fresh water to boil and simmer to cook for at least 2 hours. In this method, do not strain the cooking water from the cooked beans because you already strained and discarded unwanted sugar from beans before cooking.

Omit salt at the beginning of boiling process because some beans will harden outside and not cook inside .Little salt can be added when beans are almost ready. Remove beans and use them for your favorite secondary recipes. Cooked beans increases in size by two, (one cup raw yields two cooked).

Cooking dry maize

When maize dries it dehydrate (loose water) we need to re hydrate or add water back into the maize so it can cook easy (conduct heat).Rinse the maize to remove dust and soil. Soak dry maize just like beans (over night 8 to 10 hrs) or quick soaking (bring to boil and set aside for two hrs). Boil the maize to cook for about 2 hours. Cooked maize increases in size by two, (one cup yields two cooked).

Cooking dry maize and dry beans together (boiling Githeri)

To cook maize and beans together (githeri for 6) measure 1 cup of dry maize to 2 cup of dry beans. Soak the beans and maize **together**. Rinse and add fresh water and boil *githeri* for 2 hrs. (You are in control; check, add or reduce minutes accordingly)

Tips and variation

While boiling, keep the pot open and maintain the water above bean for about 1 hour, then cover the pot and let its steam and simmer without adding more water for the next 1 hour. This will let your beans boil and steam at the same time .By the time the food is ready your water should have reduced to less than half original level. This ensures you do not have too much liquid in the githeri. We are avoiding having to discard excess liquid.

Frying fish- fillet

Prepare both the fish and the pan. Prepare the frying pan by heating to medium high .Add a thin film of cooking oil. Do not fry wet fish .Season the fish then and dust fish lightly with some flour.

 Fish should not be too cold before placing on the pan .Cut your fillet to almost equal in sizes and in thickness .If you have a small pan or you are cooking allot of fish, cook them in bunches.

Do not overload the pan or the pan will cool down and cause the outer skin not quickly harden; and the juice will come out and ruin the quality. No fish should be placed on top of the other while frying.

Do not pull the fish off the pan in order to turn it. Fish will stick on the pan in the beginning but it will release the pan as soon as the outer skin hardens making it easier to turn.

Turn both sides to get the color you like then reduce the heat to medium low allow fish to cook fully. After you get the color you like it take just 3 to 5 additional minutes to fully cook inside depending on the size of the fillet.

Cooking Rice

Choosing rice

There are Hundreds types of rice. We can group them into 5, **long grain, short grain, parboiled and brown rice.**

Long grain cooks fluffy but some brands may mush if boiled for long before steaming. Thai Jasmine, Indian Basmati and Kenyan basmati rice has that sensational popcorn aroma .Basmati cooks fluffy and remains firm even when boiling water is slightly used in excess. Jasmine rice is softer; use less water for best quality and to avoid getting mushy.

Short grain cook sticky and are good for curtain dishes like rice pudding, soups, Italian Rice Risotto or sushi stuffing. The stickiness in short grain rice is considered best for the amazing Japanese art of chopstick dinning.

Parboiled does not mean the rice is ready cooked. However, it is a different method of processing rice grain so as nutrients are not lost while milling. The Nutrients on the outer skin are pushed inside the rice grain and then outer brown skin is removed. Amongst many marvels, America uses this method to offer her people nonstick white rice; rich with nutrients as brown rice.

Brown rice Brown rice is whole rice with outer skin. It is regarded more nutritious and has fiber. Allow brown rice to cook a little longer (10 minutes more).

Cooking rice

Rice has two primary cooking methods. In the first method, Boil the water, add salt spoonful oil to reduce sticking, rinse and add rice to steam for 7 to 8 minutes. Use the ratio of 1 cup of rice to 2 cups water, which yields 4 servings cooked rice. I prefer this method for boiling plain rice.

In the second option, Sautee/fry flavor vegetable like onions garlic ginger or for about 5 minutes. Add tomatoes and meat and other spices *(Pilau or briani masala)* Add rice then water or stock. Add salt or seasoning, bring to boil. Reduce heat to low. Cover the pot and steam for about 20 minutes. The liquid should be 1 cup for about 2 cups water for 4 servings. I prefer this method for pilau and briani

How to make Fruit Smoothie-General

Part 1

Start with basic liquid: Put Basic liquid in the puree machine, enough to cover the blade. Put either: Water, milk, yoghurt, coconut milk or juice.

Part 2

Build up the body: Add a ripened banana. Banana is commonly used to give smoothie its smooth texture.

Part 3

Add flavors: ice cream or juice. Enhance with extra nutrients if you like (protein powder, nuts, more juice or more fruits).

Part 4

Make it icy cold. Add crushed ice, select blender or puree and turn on the blender. You can add more liquid if needed to make a slow smooth flowing liquid. If you do not have the ice, you can lightly freeze all ingredients except part 1 before blending.

Use of Herbs, seasoning & marinades

Herbs: Herbs are fresh leafy parts of plants used to flavor food. There are two types of herbs: Strong and delicate. Strong herbs can withstand heat. Examples of strong herbs are rosemary leaves. Bay leaves, dill, mint, sage, parsley, marjoram and sage.

Delicate herbs cannot withstand long cooking .They lose some strength .They are best added at the last moment unless they are part of marinades. Examples of delicate herbs are dhania, spring onions, tarragon and basil.

Spices: Spices are woody bark, root or seed. They have stronger and sharp flavor than herbs .They are used in much smaller quantity than herbs. Examples of spices are black pepper, cinnamon, ginger powder, cloves, saffron, vanilla, cumin, and cardamom and mustard seeds.

*Seasoning :*Seasoning is a mixture of both spices and herbs .They are commercially put together for consumer ease of use for example; Royco, Knorr cubes, poultry seasoning, fish seasoning ,Italian seasoning and seasoned salt.

Marinades: Marinating is a process of soaking tough meat in acidic flavored liquid so as to soften it and give it more flavors. Marinades use acidic power to penetrate and soften tough meat. Marinade should include "edible" acidic item like lemon juice, vinegar herbs and spices. Add salt when ready to cook. Salt added before causes the meat to lose juice (osmosis).

Cooking tasks flow

When cooking, practice the art of cooking where you mentally can see your end product. Prepare first items which can be refrigerated like salad and fruit salad followed by cooking items that take long time to cook like stew followed by starch followed by fresh cooked vegetables .

Concluding Remarks on Nature's Fitness lifestyle

Winston S. Churchill said, "Healthy citizens are the greatest asset any country can have". Fitness lifestyle generates a set of healthy discipline. This commitment has catalytic positive influence to an improved quality of life.

This coaching is not for competitive sports. Each one of us was freely created but we have a stewardship duty to nature our bodies .This coaching is for everyone whose goal is to naturally maintain a healthy weight, have fun and enjoy the benefits associated with exercise.

When preventable health issues happens 5, 10 or 40 years later, often times they happen as though the outcome was unavoidable. Exercise and diet is the best nature's pharmacy that can prevent some health battles 5, 10 or 40 years before they occur.

Today you can take charge of your fitness. Your family and community can count on you to continue being a productive and a great asset that you are by living a nature's fitness lifestyle 24 hours a day.

Coaching References

- Republic of Kenya, National Nutrition Action Plan 2012-2017

- Kenya bureau of standards quality assurance and inspection policy.

- Kenya Utalii college food production procedures notes.

- Zambia Food security research project (FSRP)

- US bureau of labor statistics, social security administration physical exertion requirements.

- USDA 2015 dietary guidelines for American.

- World Health Organization (WHO) fact sheet on food safety

- Glycemic Index Foundation; University of Sydney Australia: List of Glycemic Index for Foods

- Nutrition Concepts and Medical Nutrition Therapy, 2012 by ANFP®

- Advanced Sports Nutrition (2nd Edition) By Dan Benardot, PhD, RD, FASM.

- NSW Health, Nutrition & Pain, Community Information Series, Hunter Integrated Pain Service; 2005.

- Moore, Dalley 4th edition. Clinically Oriented Anatomy. Lippincott Williams & Wilkins. 1999

- Deurenberg P, Westrate JA, Seidell JC. Body mass index as a measure of body fatness: age and sex prediction formulas. Brit J Nutr. 1991; 65: 105-14.